MW00897813

75 NURSE CHEAT SHEETS
for Students & New Grad Nurses

by Aaron Reed, MSN, CRNA

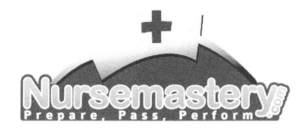

THANK YOU FOR STUDYING WITH US!

NURSEMASTERY.COM

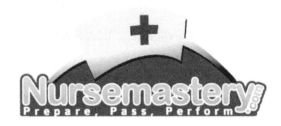

CHECKOUT:

"NCLEX REVIEW" APP
1000 NCLEX QUESTIONS eBOOK
SIGN UP FOR QUESTION OF THE DAY
twitter
youtube
facebook

FREE GIFT!

At NurseMastery.com/downloads

or

Click the link for over 75 free NCLEX questions:

LINK TO FREE NCLEX QUESTION PDF

PREVIEW...

Age	Initial Defib 2 J/kg	Repeat Defib x1 4 J/kg	Repeat Defib x2 8 J/kg	Cardio-Version 0.5-2 J/kg	Fluid Challenge 10 mL/kg
Preterm	3 J	6 J	12 J	1-3 J	15 mL
Term	7 J	14 J	28 J	2-7 J	35 mL
6 mo	14 J	28 J	56 J	4-14 J	140 mL
1 yr	20 J	40 J	80 J	5-20 J	200 mL
3 yr	30 J	60 J	120 J	8-30 J	300 mL
6 yr	40 J	80 J	160 J	10-40 J	400 mL
8 yr	50 J	100 J	200 J	13-50 J	500 mL
10 yr	60 J	120 J	240 J	15-60 J	600 mL
11 yr	70 J	140 J	280 J	18-70 J	700 mL
12 yr	80 J	160 J	320 J	20-80 J	800 mL
14 yr	90 J	180 J	360 J	23-90 J	900 mL

PREVIEW...

STAGE	FEATURES	INTERVENTIONS
I	Intact skin, painful, firm, cooler or warmer than surrounding skin, nonblanchable erythema	No dressing, protect from friction and shear forces, monitor regularly, relieve pressure, monitor frequently
II	Partial-thickness loss of epidermis or dermis, appears as abrasion, blister or shallow crater w/o slough or bruising	Dressing to keep bed evenly moist, keep surrounding skin intact & dry, loosely pack wound bed to remove excess moisture and for protection
III	Full-thickness, eschar & necrosis, subcutaneous tissue involvement, deep crater w/o undermining	Dressing to keep bed moist, surrounding tissue dry/intact, debride eschar/necrotic tissue surgically, wet-to-dry dress, mechanically, or irrigation
IV	Full-thickness, eschar, slough, necrosis, damage to muscle/bone, sinus tracts & undermining	Dressing to keep bed moist, surrounding tissue dry/intact, remove necrosis, explore undermining, control bleeding after sharp debridement then resume moist dressings

Boring Disclaimer Stuff...

As with all forms of science, nursing is a work in progress. What is taken as common knowledge today, may well be proven wrong tomorrow. Such is the nature of the scientific process. With this in mind, we stress that the information contained in this book is for the sole purpose of preparing for and mastering nursing board examinations. The information has been thoroughly reviewed and put forth with the intention of disseminating up to date knowledge and known best practices at the time of publishing. The content is not intended as a substitute for the medical advice of physicians or proper nursing training. Given the nature of this subject matter, we cannot guarantee the absence of error or promise scholastic success or clinical aptitude. All contents of this book are not to be construed as endorsements of practice or prescribed therapy for any specific clinical situation. The information to follow reflects the author's, publisher's, and all other involved party's understanding of study strategies regarding registered nursing didactic application.

We abjure any responsibility of incorrect content, consequences of enacting therapies contained within, liability to any party for any loss, damage, or disruption caused by errors or omissions, whether such errors or omissions result from negligence, accident, or any other cause. We encourage the reader to clarify any points with outside sources and consult the national standards according to your profession's governing practice body.

About the Author

started as a Respiratory Therapist in Kansas City, Missouri before attending Baker University in Kansas for
ndergraduate nursing. My first job was in the medical ICU at the University of Colorado Hospital. After practicing for
everal years I decided to attend the University of Pennsylvania in Philadelphia for Nurse Anesthesia School. I have
racticed Nurse Anesthesia in both North Carolina and the Chicago area. I have taught nursing school, performed
ursing NCLEX board symposiums, and practiced Nurse Anesthesia.

ly wife, Kristin, and I enjoy endurance sports, traveling abroad, and backpacking in Colorado. Kristin attended Baker &
enn with me and has practiced at UCH as well as North Carolina. We love education and strive to share what we know.

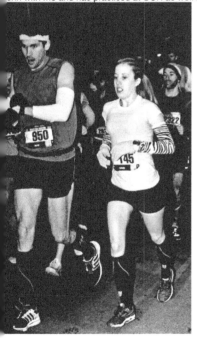

TABLE OF CONTENTS

ABBREVIATIONS

ABBREVIATION	MEANING
AED	Automated external defibrillator
ABG	Arterial blood gas
a.c.	Before a meal
ACTH	Adrenocorticotropic hormone
a.d.	Right ear (auris dextra)
ADH	Antidiuretic hormone
ADHD	Att.-deficit hyperactivity disorder
AF	Atrial fibrillation
A-fib	Atrial fibrillation
A-flutter	Atrial flutter
AFP	Alfa-fetoprotein
AI	Aortic insufficiency
AKA	Above-the-knee amputation
ALL	Acute lymphocytic leukemia
ALS	Amyotrophic lateral sclerosis
ALT	Alanine aminotransferase
AMA	Against medical advice
AMB	Ambulate
AMI	Acute myocardial infarction
AMI	Acute mitral insufficiency

CONTINUED...

ABBREVIATIONS

ABBREVIATION	MEANING
AML	Acute myelogenous leukemia
amp	Ampule/amputation
AMS	Altered mental status
AP	Anteroposterior
ARC	AIDS-related complex
ARDS	Adult resp. distress syndrome
ARF	Acute renal failure
AS	Aortic stenosis
ASA	Aspirin
a.u.	Both ears
BBB	Bundle branch block
BC	Blood cultures
BID	Twice daily
BKA	Below-the-knee amputation
BLE	Bilateral lower extremities
BM	Bowel movement
BMP	Basic metabolic panel
BPH	Benign prostatic hypertrophy
BRB	Bright red blood

CONTINUED...

ABBREVIATIONS

ABBREVIATION	MEANING
BRBPR	Bright red blood per rectum
BS	Blood sugar, bowel/breath sounds
BSA	Body surface area
BSO	Bilateral salpingo-oopherectomy
BUE	Bilateral upper extremities
BUN	Blood urea nitrogen
Bx	Biopsy
C̆	With
C&S	Culture and sensitivity
Ca	Calcium
CABG	Coronary artery bypass graft
CAD	Coronary artery disease
cap	Capsule
CBC	Complete blood count
CC	Chief complaint
cc	Cubic centimeter
CCU	Cardiac care unit
CF	Cystic fibrosis
CHD	Congenital heart disease
CHF	Congestive heart disease
CK	Creatinine kinase
CLL	Chronic lymphocytic leukemia
CML	Chronic myelocytic leukemia

CONTINUED...

ABBREVIATIONS

ABBREVIATIONS	MEANING
cm	Centimeter
CMP	Complete blood count
CMV	Cytomegalovirus
CN	Cranial nerve
CNS	Central nervous system
c/o	Complains of
CO	Cardiac output
COPD	Chronic obst. pulm. Disease
CP	Cerebral palsy/Chest pain
CPAP	Cont. positive airway press.
CPK	Creatinine phosphokinase
CRF	Chronic renal failure
CRP	C-reactive protein
CSF	Cerebrospinal fluid
CT	Computed tomography
CV	Cardiovascular
CVA	Cerebrovascular accident
CVP	Central venous pressure
CXR	Chest x-ray
D&C	Dilation & curettage
D5W	Dextrose 5% in water
DC	Discontinue/Discharge
DDx	Differential diagnosis

CONTINUED...

ABBREVIATIONS

ABBREVIATIONS	MEANING
DI	Diabetes insipidus
DJD	Degenerative joint disease
DKA	Diabetic ketoacidosis
DM	Diabetes mellitus
DNR	Do not resuscitate
DOA	Dead on arrival
DOB	Date of birth
DOE	Dyspnea on exertion
DPI	Dry powder inhaler
DRG	Diagnosis related group
DTR	Deep tendon reflex
DT's	Delirium tremens
DVT	Deep vein thrombosis
Dx	Diagnosis
EBL	Estimated blood loss
ECG	Electrocardiogram
ECHO	Echocardiogram
ECT	Electroconvulsive therapy
ED	Emergency department
EEG	Electroencephalogram
EENT	Eyes, ears, nose, throat
EMG	Electromyogram

CONTINUED...

ABBREVIATIONS

ABBREVIATIONS	MEANING
ENT	Ears, nose, throat
EOM	Extraocular movement
ESLD	End-stage liver disease
ESRD	End-stage renal disease
ETOH	Ethanol/alcohol
ETT	Endotracheal tube
FBS	Fasting blood sugar
FEV	Forced expiratory volume
FEV1	Forced exp. Volume in 1 sec.
FFP	Fresh frozen plasma
FIO2	Fraction of inspired oxygen
FROM	Full range of motion
FSH	Follicle stimulating hormone
F/U	Follow-up
FUO	Fever of unknown origin
FVC	Forced vital capacity
Fx	Fracture
GC	Gonorrhea
GERD	Gastroesophageal reflux
GFR	Glomerular filtration rate
GH	Growth hormone
GI	Gastrointestinal

CONTINUED...

ABBREVIATIONS

ABBREVIATIONS	MEANING
g	Gram
GN	Glomerular nephritis
gr	Grain
GSW	Gunshot wound
gtt	Drops
GTT	Glucose tolerance test
GU	Genitourinary
GYN	Gynecology
HA	Headache
HBV	Hepatitis B virus
HCT	Hematocrit
HCO3	Bicarbonate
HCTZ	Hydrochlorothiazide
HDL	High-density lipoprotein
HF	Heart failure
Hg	Mercury
Hgb	Hemoglobin
HPI	History of present illness
HPV	Human papilloma virus
HR	Heart rate
HSR	Herpes simplex virus
HTN	Hypertension
Hx	History

CONTINUED...

ABBREVIATIONS

ABBREVIATIONS	MEANING
I&D	Incision and drainage
I&O	Intake and output
IBD	Inflammatory bowel disease
IBS	Irritable bowel disease
ID	Infectious disease
Ig	Immunoglobulin
IHD	Ischemic heart disease
IM	Intramuscular
insp.	Inspiratory
IOP	Intraocular pressure
IP	Intraperitoneal
IPPB	Intermittent pos. press. Breath
IT	Intrathecal
IUD	Intrauterine device
IVC	Inferior vena cava
IVDA	Intravenous drug abuse
IVP	Intravenous pyelogram
IVPB	Intravenous piggyback
IVSD	Intraventricular septal defect
JRA	Juvenile rheumatoid arthritis
JVD	Jugular vein distention
Kg	Kilogram

CONTINUED...

ABBREVIATIONS

ABBREVIATIONS	MEANING
KCL	Potassium chloride
KUB	Kidney, ureters, bladder
KVO	Keep vein open
L	Liter
L/m	Liters per minute
L&D	Labor and delivery
LAD	Left anterior descending
LAN	Lymphadenopathy
LBBB	Left bundle branch block
LDH	Lactose dehydrogenase
LDL	Low-density lipoprotein
LES	Lower esophageal sphincter
LFT	Liver function test
LH	Luteinizing hormone
lmp	Last menstrual period
LLE	Left lower extremity
LOC	Loss of consciousness
LP	Lumbar puncture
LUE	Left upper extremity
LUQ	Left upper quadrant
LV	Left ventricle
LVEDP	L. vent. end-diastolic press.
LVH	Left ventricular hypertrophy

CONTINUED...

ABBREVIATIONS

ABBREVIATIONS	MEANING
MAO	Monoamine oxidase
MAP	Mean arterial pressure
MBT	Maternal blood pressure
mcg	Microgram
MDI	Metered dose inhaler
mEq	Milliequivalent
MCH	Mean corpuscular hemoglobin
MCHC	Mean corpuscular hgb conc.
MCV	Mean corpuscular volume
MI	Mitral insufficiency
MI	Myocardial infarction
mL	Milliliter
MM	Multiple myeloma
mmHg	Millimeters mercury
MR	Mitral regurgitation
MRI	Magnetic resonance imaging
MRSA	Methicillin-resistant staph aur.
MS	Mental status/Mitral stenosis
MS	Multiple sclerosis
MVA	Motor vehicle accident
Na	Sodium
NC	Nasal cannula
NCAT	Normocephalic, atraumatic

CONTINUED...

ABBREVIATIONS

ABBREVIATIONS	MEANING
Neb	Nebulizer
NG	Nasogastric
NICU	Neonatal intensive care unit
NIDDM	Non-insulin dependent DM
NKA	No known allergies
NKDA	No know drug allergies
NPH	Neutral protamine hagedorn
NPO	Nothing by mouth
NRB	Non-rebreather mask
NS	Normal saline
NSR	Normal sinus rhythm
NT	Nasothracheal/nontender
NTG	Nitroglycerin
N/V	Nausea & vomiting
OA	Osteoarthritis
OB	Obstetrics
O.D.	Right eye
OM	Otitis media
ORIF	Open reduce, internal fixation
OTC	Over the counter
OS	Left eye
OU	Each eye
oz.	Ounce

CONTINUED...

ABBREVIATIONS

ABBREVIATIONS	MEANING
PA	Pulmonary artery
PA	Posterior anterior
PAB	Premature atrial beat
PAC	Premature atrial contraction
PAP	Pulmonary artery pressure
PAWP	Pulm. artery wedge pressure
pc	After meals
PCN	Penicillin
PCP	Pneumocystis carinii pneum.
PDA	Patent ductus arteriosus
PE	Pulmonary embolism
PE	Pleural effusion
PEEP	Positive end expiratory press.
PFT	Pulmonary function test
PID	Pelvic inflammatory disease
PIP	Peak inspiratory pressure
PMH	Past medical history
PMI	Point of maximum impulse
PO	Per os, by mouth
PPD	Packs per day
PR	Per rectum
PRBC	Packed red blood cell
PRN	As needed

CONTINUED...

ABBREVIATIONS

ABBREVIATIONS	MEANING
PS	Pulmonic stenosis
PSA	Prostatic specific antigen
PT	Prothrombin time
PTA	Prior to admission
PTH	Parathyroid hormone
PTT	Partial thromboplastin time
PUD	Peptic ulcer disease
PVB	Preventricular beat
PVC	Premature vent. contraction
PVD	Peripheral vascular disease
q	Every "#" hours/minutes/etc.
Q	Perfusion
qd	Daily
qh	Hourly
qid	Four times daily
qod	Every other day
RA	Rheumatoid arthritis
RA	Right atrium
RAD	Right axis deviation
RBBB	Right bundle branch block
RBC	Red blood cell
RDA	Recommend daily allowance
REM	Rapid eye movement

CONTINUED...

ABBREVIATIONS

ABBREVIATIONS	MEANING
RF	Renal/respiratory failure
RFT	Renal function test
RHD	Rheumatic heart disease
RLL	Right lower lobe
RLQ	Right lower quadrant
RML	Right middle lobe
R/O	Rule out
ROM	Range of motion
ROS	Review of systems
RR	Respiratory rate
RRR	Regular rate and rhythm
RT	Radiation/respiratory therapy
RUL	Right upper lobe
RUQ	Right upper quadrant
RV	Residual volume
RVH	Right ventricular hypertrophy
Rx	Prescription
š	Without (sans)
S1, S2, S3, S4	1st, 2nd, 3rd, 4th heart sounds
SBO	Small-bowel obstruction
Subcut	Subcutaneously
SCM	Sternocleidomastoid
SL	Sublingual

CONTINUED...

ABBREVIATIONS

ABBREVIATIONS	MEANING
SLE	Systemic lupus erythematous
SOA	Short of air
SOB	Short of breath
SpO2	Pulse oximeter O2 saturation
s/p	Status post
s/s	Signs and symptoms
STAT	Immediately
STI	Sexually transmitted infection
SVC	Superior vena cava
Sx	Surgery/symptom/suction
T	Temperature
T3	Triiodothyronine
T4	Tetraiodothyronine
T&A	Tonsillectomy, adenoidectomy
T&C	Type and cross
Tab	Tablet
TAH	Total abdominal hysterectomy
TB	Tuberculosis
TBA	To be announced
TBI	Traumatic brain injury
Td	Tetanus-diphtheria toxoid
TFT	Thyroid function test
TIA	Transient ischemic attack

CONTINUED

ABBREVIATIONS

ABBREVIATIONS	MEANING
TID	Three times daily
TLC	Total lung capacity
TMJ	Temporomandibular joint
TO	Telephone order
tPA	Tissue plasminogen activator
TPN	Total parenteral nutrition
TSH	Thyroid-stimulating hormone
TT	Thrombin time
TURP	Transurethral resection proc.
TVH	Transvaginal hysterectomy
Tx	Treatment
UA	Urinalysis
UC	Ulcerative colitis
UE	Upper extremity
URI	Upper respiratory infection
US	Ultrasound
UTI	Urinary tract infection
VA	Visual acuity
VC	Vital capacity
VD	Venereal disease
VF	Ventricular fibrillation
VO	Verbal order
VRE	Vanco. resistant enterococcus

CONTINUED...

ABBREVIATIONS

ABBREVIATIONS	MEANING
VSD	Ventricular septal defect
VSS	Vital signs stable
VT	Ventricular tachycardia
w/a	While awake
WB	Whole blood
WBC	White blood cells
WN	Well nourished
WNL	Within normal limits
WOB	Work of breathing
WPW	Wolff-Parkinson White
W/O	Without
WTD	Wet-to-dry
W/U	Work up
x	Times per "X"
XM	Cross match
YO	Years old
Zn	Zinc

ABG ANALYSIS

PARAMETER	NORMAL VALUE	NORMAL RANGE	MEANING
pH	7.4	7.35-7.40	Acid-base status of blood pH >7.45 = alkalosis pH<7.35 = acidosis
PaCO2	40 mmHg	35-45 mmHg	Carbon dioxide <35=Hyperventilation >45=Resp. Acidosis or hypermetabolic state
PaO2	100 mmHg	80-100mmHg	Partial Pressure Oxygen <80=Hypoxemia <65=Give supplemental O2
HCO3	24 mEq/L	22-26 mEq/L	Bicarbonate concentration <22=Metabolic acidosis >26=Metabolic alkalosis
BE	0	+2 to -2	Amount of acid/base that must be added for pH 7.4. <-2=Metabolic acidosis >+2=Metabolic alkalosis
Hgb	14 g/dL	12-18 g/dL	Hemoglobin:O2 carrying component of blood. <9=Need bloodTransfusion
O2 content	20 ml O2/100ml	16-22 ml O2/100ml	Total volume of dissolved O2 + O2 bound to Hgb per 100ml of blood.
SaO2	98%	>95%	Saturation level of oxygen in Hgb. <92%= Give O2.
COHb	0	<2%	Carbon Monoxide bound Hgb. from smoke hindering O2 carrying capacity
MetHb	0	<2%	Hgb unable to bind O2 from poison.(Methemoglobin.)

ABG INTERPRETATION

INTERPRETATION	PH	PaCO2	HCO3
RESPIRATORY ACIDOSIS			
Acute	↓	↑	N
Chronic/compensated	N	↑	↑
Chronic with acute	↓	↑	↑
RESPIRATORY ALKALOSIS			
Acute	↑	↓	N
Compensated/chronic	N	↓	↓
METABOLIC ACIDOSIS			
Acute	↓	N	↓
Compensated	N	↓	↓
METABOLIC ALKALOSIS			
Acute	↑	N	↑
Compensated	N	↑	↑

ACLS BRADYCARDIA

Assess clinical condition: hypotension, altered mental status
Heart rate usually <60 bpm
Identify & treat underlying causes
Maintain airway & assist breathing prn
O2, pulse ox, BP, IV, cardiac monitor, 12-lead ECG

UNREMITTING BRADYCARDIA
- Atropine 0.5 mg IV push, q3-5 min (max 3 mg)
- Transcutaneous pacing
- Dopamine 2-10 mcg/kg/min IV
- Epinephrine 2-10 mcg/min

ACLS STROKE

Activate Emergency Response & Stroke Team
ABC's, Vital Signs, Oxygen
Obtain time of symptom onset
IV, Labs, Check glucose, H&P, Neuro Exam
NIH Stroke & Canadian Neuro Scale
Emergency brain CT & 12-lead ECG

CT SCAN WITH HEMORRHAGE
Consult neurologist or neurosurgeon
Stroke or hemorrhage pathway
Reduce BP, antiepileptics, FFP
Reverse warfarin (Vit K), Reverse heparin (protamine)

CT SCAN WITH ISCHEMIC STROKE
Exclude patient if stroke symptoms >3-4.5 hours or ASA

FIBRINOLYTIC THERAPY
rtPa if no anticoagulants or antiplatelet for 24 hrs.

ACLS TACHYCARDIA

Assess clinical condition: hypotension, altered mental status
Heart rate >150 bpm
Identify & treat underlying causes (H's & T's)
Maintain airway, assist breathing prn
O2, pulse ox, BP, IV, cardiac monitor, 12-lead ECG

UNREMITTING SYMPTOMATIC TACHYCARDIA
- Synchronized Cardioversion
    - Narrow regular: 50-100J
    - Narrow irregular: 120-200J bi/200J monophasic
    - Wide regular: 100J
    - Wide irregular: defibrillation unsynchronized
- Narrow Regular
    - Adenosine 6 mg rapid IV push, then 12 mg prn

STABLE TACHYCARDIA
- Vagal maneuvers
- Beta-blockers, Calcium channel blockers
- Expert consultation

ACLS ACUTE CORONARY SYNDROME

IMMEDIATE TREATMENT
- O2, titrate SpO2 > 92%
- Aspirin 160-325 mg
- Nitroglycerin Sublingual/Spray
- Morphine IV

ASSESSMENT
- Vitals, SpO2, IV, H&P
- Perform Fibrinolytic checklist
- Draw troponin, CK-MB, electrolytes, coags
- Chest X-ray, ECG

ST ELEVATION (STEMI) OR LBBB
- Onset <12 hrs. = *Fibrinolysis*, *PCI* (balloon inflation), ACE-Inhibitor, Statin, Beta-blocker, Clopidogrel, Heparin

ST DEPRESSION OR T-WAVE INVERSION (NSTEMI)
- Nitroglycerin, Heparin, Clopidogrel, Beta-blocker, Glycoprotein IIb/IIIa inhibitor

ACLS CARDIAC ARREST

CPR, O2, MONITOR, DEFIBRILLATOR

VENTRICULAR FIBRILLATION/V. TACHYCARDIA (VF/VT)
- SHOCK
- CPR for 2 minutes
- IV/IO Access
- EPINEPHRINE 1 mg q3-5 min. or
  - →VASOPRESSIN 40 units for 1st or 2nd Epi dose
  - →Consider Advanced Airway & Capnography
- AMIODARONE 300 mg (2nd dose 150mg)
  - →Check rhythm, shock VF/VT after 2 min CPR

ASYSTOLE/PULSELESS ELECTRICAL ACIVITY (PEA)
- CPR for 2 minutes
- IV/IO access
- EPINEPHRINE 1 mg q3-5 min. or
  - →VASOPRESSIN 40 unit for 1st or 2ns Epi dose
  - →Consider Advanced Airway & Capnography
  - →Check rhythm, shock VF/VT after 2 min CPR

TREAT REVERSIBLE CAUSES (H's & T's)
Hypovolemia, hypoxia, hydrogen ion, hypo/hyperkalemia, hypothermia
Tension pneumothorax, tamponade, toxins, thrombosis

ACLS POST CARDIAC ARREST

★RETURN OF SPONTANEOUS CIRCULATION (ROSC)★

ENHANCE VETILATION & OXYGENATION
- Maintain SpO2 > 95%
- Advanced airway and capnography as needed
  ➜Hyperventilation ⬇'s cerebral blood flow!

TISSUE PRESERVATION (CEREBRAL & CARDIAC)
- Consider Therapeutic Hypothermia
- PCI (percutaneous coronary intervention)
- Glycemic Control

TREAT HYPOTENSION
- Normal Saline 1-2 L IV bolus
- Vasopressor drips (epi/dopa/norepi)
- Treat reversible causes
- 12-lead ECG

ADMIT TO CRITICAL CARE

ADMIT NOTE

ADMIT: Unit, floor, room, medical service, attending
DIAGNOSES: Primary, secondary, chronic, acute
CONDITION: Stable, fair, serious, critical, undetermined
VITALS: Frequency (q2 hrs., q shift, routine)
DIET: NPO, regular, low sodium, diabetic, clears, liquid
ACTIVITY: Bed rest, up to chair, ad lib, ambulate BID
MEDS: Pain, insulin, antibiotics, anticoagulants, ppi
ALLERGIES: NKA, medications, foods, tape, dye
I&O: IV fluid rate, foley, nasogastric tube, strict
LABS: ABG, CBC, CMP, coags, EKG, X-rays, CT/MRI
MONITORS: Swan, CVP, NIBP, arterial line, telemetry, SpO2
RESPIRATORY: ETT, NC, incentive spirometry, CPAP
DRESSINGS: TED hose, surgical wounds, change frequency

APGAR

	0	1	2
APPEARANCE	Entire body blue or pale	Pink body with blue extremities	Entire body pink
PULSE	Absent	<100 bpm	>100bpm
GRIMACE	No response	Grimace or slight cry	Cough, sneeze, cry
ACTIVITY	Limp, motionless	Some flexion	Active movement
RESPIRATIONS	Absent	Slow, irregular	Strong, crying

NOTE: Test is generally done at 1 and 5 minutes after birth, and may be repeated later if the score is and remains low.

- 8-10 = Considered normal
- 5-7 = O2 mask (mech. vent. if needed), stimulation
- 3-6 = Mechanical vent mask, intubate if needed
- <2 = Intubation, chest compression if HR < 60 bpm
- HR < 100 bpm = Positive pressure ventilation

ARTIFICIAL AIRWAY, ENDOTRACHEAL TUBE, & LARYNGOSCOPE BY AGE

AGE	ETT INTERNAL DIAMETER (MM)	LARYNGOSCOPE BLADE SIZE	SUCTION CATHER (French)
Newborn <1000 g 1000-2000 g 2000-3000 g >3000 g	2.5 3 3.5 3.5-4	Miller 0 Miller 0 Miller 1 Miller 1	5 6 6-8 6-8
6 months	3-4	Miller 1	6-8
1 year	4-4.5	Wis-hipple 1.5 Miller 1	8
2-3 years	4.5-5	Wis-hipple 1.5 Miller 2	8
4-7 years	5-6	Miller 2	8-10
8-10 years	6-6.5	Miller 2	10
12 years	7	Miller 2	10
15 years	7-7.5	Miller 2 Mac 3-4	10-12
Adult M.	7-8	Mac 3-4	14
Adult F.	7-8.5	Mac 3-4	12

BLOOD CHEMISTRY

LAB	SI Units	CONVENTIONAL
Alanine transaminase (ALT)	M: 10-40 units/L F:7-35units/L	M: 10-40 units/L F:7-35units/L
Albumin	35-48 g/L	3.5-5 g/dL
Alkaline phosphate	M: 35-145 units/L F: 25-125 units/L	M: 35-145 units/L F: 25-125 units/L
Ammonia	M: 20-75 µmol/L F: 15-65 µmol/L	M: 25-105 mcg/L F: 20-85 mcg/L
Amylase	30-110 units/L	30-110 units/L
Anion gap	8-16 mmol/l	8-16 mEq/L
Aspartate aminotransferase (AST)	M2-59: 15-40 units/L M 60-90: 20-48 u/L F 2-59: 12-35 units/L F 60-90: 10-35 u/L	15-40 units/L 20-48 units/L 12-35 units/L 10-35 units/L
Bilirubin, conjugated	< 5 µmol/L	< 0.3 mg/dL
Bilirubin, total	5-20 µmol/L	0.3-1.2 mg/dL
Calcium	2.1-2.6 mmol/L	8-10 mg/dL
Calcium, ionized	1.1-1.3 mmol/dL	4.6-5.3 mg/dL
Carbon dioxide (CO2)	21-28 mmol/L	22-26 mE1/dL
Chloride (Cl)	95-106 mmol/L	95-106 mEq/L
Cholesterol (HDL)	> 0.9 mmol/L	> 40 mg/dL
Cholesterol (LDL)	< 2.6 mmol/L	< 100 mg/dL

CONTINUED...

BLOOD CHEMISTRY

LAB	SI UNITS	CONVENTIONAL
Cholesterol, total	< 5.2 mmol/L	< 200 mg/dL
Cortisol	am:200-650 nmol/L pm: < 50 nmol/L	7-24 mcg/dL < 18 mcg/dL
Creatine kinase (CK)	M: 50-200 units/L F: 35-150 units/L	50-200 units/L 35-150 units/L
Creatinine	M: 50-105 µmol/L F: 45-100 µmol/L	0.6-1.2 mg/dL 0.5-1.1 mg/dL
Folate	> 5.8 nmol/L	> 2.5 ng/mL
Glucose	3.5-5.5 mmol/L	70-100 mg/dL
Iron (Fe)	M: 11.5-30 µmol/L F: 10-30 µmol/L	65-170 mcg/dL 50-165 mcg/dL
LDH	90-175 units/L	90-175 units/L
Lactic acid	0.3-2.5 mmol/L	3-22 mg/dL
Lipase	3-75 units/L	3-75 units/L
Magnesium (Mg)	0.6-1.1 mmol/L	1.5-2.7 mg/dL
Osmolality	250-900 mmol/kg	250-900 mmol/kg
Phosphorus	0.8-1.5 mmol/L	2.5-4.5 mg/dL
Potassium (K)	3.5-5.0 mmol/L	3.5-5.0 mEq/L
Prealbumin	125-400 mg/L	11-40 mg/dL
Protein, total	60-80 g/L	6.0-8.0 g/dL
Sodium (Na)	135-145 mmol/L	135-145 mEq/L

CONTINUED...

BLOOD CHEMISTRY

LAB	SI UNITS	CONVENTIONAL
Thyroglobulin	0-50 mcg/L	0-50 ng/mL
Thyroid-stim. (TSH)	0.4-4.2 µIU/L	0.4-4.2 µIU/L
Thyroxin (T4), free	10-20 pmol/L	0.9-1.5 ng/dL
Thyroxin (T4), total	M: 60-135 nmol/L F: 70-145 nmol/L	4.5-10.5 mcg/dL 5.5-11.0 mcg/dL
Triglycerides	0.4-1.5 g/L	40-150 mg/dL
T3, free	4.0-7.5 mmol/L	250-475 pg/dL
Urea nitrogen (BUN)	3.0-7.5 mmol/L	8-20 mg/dL
Uric acid	M: 0.25-.45 mmol/L F: 0.14-0.4 mmol/L	4.5-7.5 mg/dL F: 2.3-6.5 mg/dL

BLOOD COMPATIBILITY

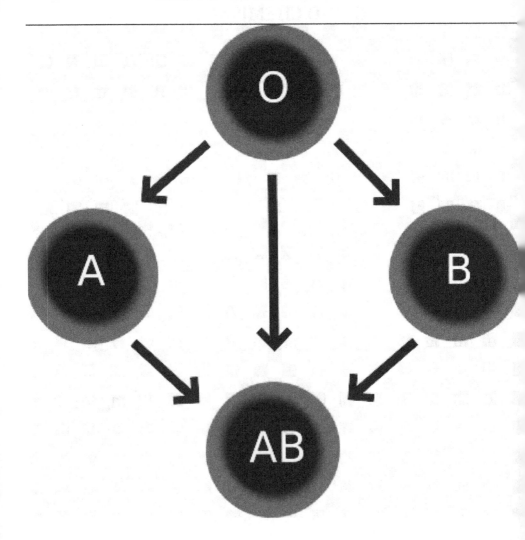

BLOOD GAS FORMULA

NAME	NORMAL VALUE	FORMULA
CaO2 O2 content of arterial blood	15-20 vol%	(hb x 1.34 x SaO2) + (PaO2 x 0.003)
CvO2 O2 content of mixed venous	12-15 vol%	(Hb x 1.34 x SvO2) + (PvO2 x 0.003)
C(a-v)O2 Artery to venous O2 content diff.	3.5-5.0 vol%	CaO2 – CvO2 Tissue oxygenation
Pa-vDO2 Partial press. artery–to-vein	50 mmHg	PaO2 – PvO2 Tissue oxygenation
PAO2	100 mmHg	(PB – PH2O) x FIO2 – (PaCO2 /0.8) *PB=Barometric press., PH20=47*
P(A-a)O2 (A-a) Alveolar-to-artery gradient	<26 mmHg (RA) <100 mmHg on FIO2 of 100%	PAO2 – PaO2 Gradient shows diffusion deficit/shunt
PaO2 Artery partial pressure of O2	80-100 mmHg	Lab value

BLOOD PRODUCTS

BLOOD PRODUCT	INFO	INDICATION
Packed Red Blood Cells (match ABO/Rh)	No clotting factors, 80% plasma. Leukocyte reduced prevent febrile reaction	Increase O2 carrying capacity. If Hbg < 8 mg/dL.
Platelets (match ABO/Rh/HLA)	Platelets only. 1 unit ↑'s count by 5,000.	Prevent bleeding with ↓ platelet or coagulopathy.
Fresh Frozen Plasma (match ABO)	Plasma & clotting factors.	Replace factors after large transfusions or Coumadin OD.
Cryoprecipitate (prefer match ABO)	Clotting factors & fibrinogen.	Bleeding r/t DIC, hemophilia, fibrinogen deficiency.
Factor IX concentrate	Risk hepatitis d/t pooled donors	Treat hemophilia B
Factor VIII conc.	Heat-treated ↓ risk of Hep/HIV	Treat hemophilia A
Whole Blood (match ABO/Rh)	Contains all blood products. Rarely used.	Exsanguinating patient, massive transfusion.

BLS ALGORITHM

UNRESPONSIVE, ALTERED RESPIRATIONS
Activate Emergency Response System
Get AED/Defibrillator

PULSE

Give 1 breath every 5-6 seconds
Check pulse every 2 minutes

NO PULSE

Begin CPR 100 comp/min
30 compression:2 breaths

AED/DEFIBRILLATOR ARRIVES

SHOCKABLE RHYTHM
Give 1 shock
Resume CPR for 2 min.

NON-SHOCKABLE RHYTHM
Resume CPR for 2 min.

★RECHECK RHYTHM EVERY 2 MINUTES & REPEAT★

BODY MASS INDEX & BODY SURFACE AREA

BODY SURFACE AREA (BSA) (m^2)

Square root of (height [in] x weight [lb.]) / 3131
or
Square root of (height [cm] x weight [kg]) / 3600

Example
BSA of 70-inch-tall, 170-lb. male = 1.95 m^2

BODY MASS INDEX (BMI)

(Weight in pounds x 700) / (height in inches^2)
or
(Weight in kg) / (meters^2)

Example
BMI of 70-inch-tall, 170-lb. male = 24.4

BRADEN SCALE

	1	2	3	4
Sensory Perception	Completely Limited	Very Limited	Slightly Limited	No Impair
Moisture	Constantly Moist	Very Moist	Sometime Moist	Rarely Moist
Activity	Bedfast	Chair fast	Sometime Walks	Walks A Lot
Mobility	Completely Immobile	Very Limited	Slightly Limited	No Limit

< 9 = Severe Risk
10-12 = High Risk
13-14 = Moderate Risk
15-18 = Mild Risk

CARDIAC VOLUMES & PRESSURES

	PARAMETER	NORMAL	CALCULATION
CI	Cardiac Index	3-4.5L/min/m^2	CO/BSA
CO	Cardiac Output	4-8 L/min	HR X SV(ml) / 1000 OR VO2/(CaO2 – CvO x100)
CVP	Central Venous press.	2-8 mm Hg	Estimates right ventricle preload & volume status.
EF	Ejection Fraction	65-75%	SV / End diastolic vol.
LVP	Left Vent. Pressure	90/130 mmHg / 1-12 mmHg	Filling pressure of left ventricle.
MAP	Mean Arterial Pressure	80-100 mmHg	((Systolic BP) + (2x diastolic BP)) / 3
PAP	Pulmonary Artery Press.	15-30 mmHg / 5-15 mmHg	Pulmonary artery catheter needed.
PCWP	Pulm. Capillary Wedge Press.	4-12 mmHg	Estimates L. vent filling & preload. Equal to left atrial pressure.
RVP	Right Vent. Pressure	20-30 mmHg / 2-8 mmHg	Filling pressure of right ventricle.
SI	Stroke Index	40-60 ml/beat/m^2	SV/BSA. Cardiac function relative to body size.
SV	Stroke Vol.	50-120 ml/beat	(CO in L/m ÷ HR) x 1000
SVR	System Vascular Resistance	15-20 mmHg/L/min 1000-1600 dynes	(MAP – CVP) / CO Multiply by 80 for dynes

CARDIOVERSION, DEFIBRILLATION, & FLUID CHALLENGE

Age	Initial Defib 2 J/kg	Repeat Defib x1 4 J/kg	Repeat Defib x2 8 J/kg	Cardio-Version 0.5-2 J/kg	Fluid Challenge 10 mL/kg
Preterm	3 J	6 J	12 J	1-3 J	15 mL
Term	7 J	14 J	28 J	2-7 J	35 mL
6 mo	14 J	28 J	56 J	4-14 J	140 mL
1 yr	20 J	40 J	80 J	5-20 J	200 mL
3 yr	30 J	60 J	120 J	8-30 J	300 mL
6 yr	40 J	80 J	160 J	10-40 J	400 mL
8 yr	50 J	100 J	200 J	13-50 J	500 mL
10 yr	60 J	120 J	240 J	15-60 J	600 mL
11 yr	70 J	140 J	280 J	18-70 J	700 mL
12 yr	80 J	160 J	320 J	20-80 J	800 mL
14 yr	90 J	180 J	360 J	23-90 J	900 mL

CHEST PAIN

CAUSE	CHARACTERISTICS
Myocardial Ischemia	Sudden, crushing, radiating pain. If it occurs with exertion and is relieved by rest, it may be angina.
Pericarditis	Intermittent caused by breathing or supine. Relieved by leaning forward.
Pancreatitis	Pain in epigastric region or lower chest.
Esophageal Reflux	Burning from epigastric to throat. Aggravated lying down. Antacids help.
Pulmonary Embolism	Pleuritic chest pain & sudden dyspnea.
Thoracic Aortic dissection	Acute, searing pain, radiates to back or groin, accompanied by syncope.
Pericarditis	Constant or occasional sharp pain. Worsens with breathing and supine. Improves sitting forward.
Esophageal Rupture	Acute, severe pain with hematemesis.
Peptic Ulcer	Intermittent, radiating pain in epigastric region or radiating to right upper quadrant. Antacids or food may help.
Pleuritis	Acute pain with breathing or coughing.
Biliary Tract Disease	Right upper quadrant pain after meals.

COAGULATION STUDIES

LAB	NORMAL VALUE
Bleeding Time	2-7 minutes
Activated Clotting time (ACT)	90-130 seconds
Activated partial thromboplastin time (aPTT)	25-40 seconds
Thrombin Time	13-16 seconds
Fibrinogen	1.6-4.5 g/L *or* 200-400 mg/dl
International Normalized Ratio (INR)	1-1.3 w/o anticoagulants 2-3 with anticoagulants
Plasminogen	80-120% of plasma
Platelets	150-400 x 10^9/L
Prothrombin Time (PT)	11-13.5 seconds
Partial Thromboplastin time (PTT)	25-40 seconds

CODE DRUGS

DRUG	INDICATION	DOSE	DETAILS
Adenosine	PVST	6 mg IV rapid flush	Chest pain, BP drop, bradycardia
Amiodorone	VT, VF, AF, SVT, PSVT	300 mg IV, Wide QRS 150	Prolonged QT Hypotension
Atropine	Bradycardia	1 mg IVq3min	Myocardial demand
Calcium Chl.	Hyperkalemia Hypocalcemia	0.-1 g slowly q10 min.	Brady., asystole, or hypotension
Dextrose 50	Hypoglycemia	50ml slow IVP	Fluid overload
Dobutamine	Low CO, CHF	2-20 mcg/k/m	Tachycardia
Dopamine	↓HR, ↓BP	5-10 mcg/k/m	Myocardia demand
Epinephrine	Cardiac arrest	1mg IVP q3m	1:10k = 0.1mg/mL
Flumazenil	↓RR: Benzo's	0.2mg up to 1	Repeat q1 min.
Lidocaine	VT, VF	1mg/kg max 3	Reduce dose CHF
Mag Sulfate	VF, Torsades	1-2mg IVP	↓BP, Caution Renal
Nitroglycerin	Angina, HTN	10-20mcg/m. 0.5mg SL q5 x3	Hypotension, HA
Nor-Epi	Hypotension	2-20 mcg/min	Myocardial demand Arrhythmias
Bicarbonate	↓K, Acidosis	1 mEq/kg IVP	∅ Cardiac arrest

COLLOIDS

SOLUTION	CONTENTS	INDICATIONS
Albumin 5%	Human Plasma Protein	Rapid volume expansion & interstitial edema.
Albumin 25%	Human Plasma Protein	Mobilize interstitial edema, Low protein
6% Dextran 70 10% Dextran 40	Synthetic Colloid	Volume expansion. Mobilize edema.
Hetastarch/Hespan	Synthetic colloid	Volume expansion. Mobilize edema.

COMPLETE BLOOD COUNT

LAB	SI UNITS	CONVENTIONAL
Red blood cells (RBC)	M: 4.5-6.5 x 10^{12}/L F: 3.8-5.8 x 10^{12}/L	4.5-6.5 x 10^6cell/mm^3 3.8-5.8 x 10^6cell/mm^3
Hemoglobin (Hgb)	M: 8.4-10.9 mmol/L F: 7.4-9.9 mmol/L	13-17 g/dL 11.5-15.5 g/dL
Hematocrit (Hct)	M: 0.4-0.5 F: 0.36-0.44	40.7-50.3% 36-44.3%
Platelet	150-400 x 10^9/L	150-400 x 10^3/mm^3
Leukocyte (WBC)	5-10 x 10^9/L	5-10 x 10^3/mm^3
Erythrocyte sedimentation rate (ESR)	M: 0-15 mm/hr F: 0-25 mm/hr	0-15 mm/hr 0-25 mm/hr
Glycolated hemoglobin (HbgA1C)	4.0-7.0%	4.0-7.0%
Basophil Eosonphil Lymphocyte Monocyte Neutrophil Bands	0-0.01 x 10^9/L 0.0-0.08 x 10^9/L 0.2-0.52 x 10^9/L 0.04-0.12 x 10^9/L 0.34-0.7 x 10^9/L 0.0-0.01 x 10^9/L	0%-1% 0%-8% 20%-52% 4%-12% 34%-70% 0%-10%

CONVERSIONS

MICROGRAMS
100 mcg = 0.1 mg
1000 mcg = 1 mg

MILLIGRAMS
1 mg = 0.001 gram
100 mg = 0.1 gram = 0.0001 kg = 0.0035 oz.
1000 mg = 1.0 gram = 0.001 kg = 0.035 oz.

MILLILITERS
1 mL = 1 cc = 20 drops
30 mL = 1 cc = 28 grams
1000 mL = 1 L
1 tsp. = 5 mL
1 Tbsp. = 15 mL
1 cup = 240 mL = 0.24 liters = 8 oz.
1 pint = 474 mL = 0.47 liters = 16 oz.
1 quart = 946 mL = 0.95 liters = 32 oz.
1 gallon = 3.79 liters = 128 oz.

KILOGRAMS & POUNDS
Pounds / 2.2 = kilograms
Kilograms x 2.2 = pounds
1 lbs. = 0.45 kg = 454 grams = 16 oz.
1 kg = 2.2 lbs. = 1000 grams = 35.3 oz.

MISCELLANEOUS
1 mmHg = 1 torr = 1.36 cmH2O
torr x 1.36 = cmH2O
cmH2O / 1.36 = torr

CRANIAL NERVES

NERVE	FUNCTION	TEST
I – Olfactory	Smell	Identify smells
II – Optic	Visual acuity visual field	Visual acuity eye chart, peripherals
III – Oculomotor	Pupillary reaction	Pupils equal and reactive to light
IV – Trochlear	Eye movement	Follow finger with eyes & head still
V – Trigeminal	Facial sensation & movement	Sharp & dull sensation on face. Open mouth
VI – Abducens	Motor movement	Follow finger with eyes & head still
VII - Facial	Taste & facial movement	Smile, puff cheeks. Sweet/salty tastes
VIII – Acoustic	Hearing & balance	Finger snap. Stand feet together, eyes closed 5 seconds.
IX - Glossopharyngeal	Swallowing & voice	Swallow and say "ah"
X – Vagus	Gag reflex	Elicit gag w/ tongue blade
XI – Spinal accessory	Neck movement	Shrug & turn head against resistance
XII - Hypoglossal	Tongue motion	Stick out tongue & move side-to-side

CRYSTALLOIDS

SOLUTION	CONTENTS	INDICATIONS
Saline Solution (0.9%, 0.45, 0.25%)	Sodium & Chloride NaCl	Fluid replacement Sodium deficit
Dextrose Solution (D5W, D10W)	Dextrose in Water	Replace calories, Preserve water, Prevent dehydration, Create Na diuresis
Dextrose & Saline (D5NS, D50.45%NS)	Dextrose in Saline	Correct fluid loss Calories & Chloride Create diuresis
Lactated Ringer's	Na, Cl, K, Ca, Lactate	Replace gastric electrolytes, Dehydration, Restore fluid balance

DAILY BODY FLUIDS

FLUID	Na	K	Cl	HCO3	Volume
Salivary	10	25	10	30	500-200
Gastric	60	10	125	0	100-4000
Biliary	150	5	100	35	50-800
Pancreatic	145	5	70	120	100-800
Ileal	130	5	100	50	100-9000
Diarrheal	60	40	40	30	Fluctuates

DEEP TENDON REFLEX SCALE

0	No response (absent).
+1	Diminished or sluggish response. Reflex slight, less than normal.
+2	Normal or expected response.
+3	More brisk than expected, slightly stronger than normal response.
+4	Hyperactive and brisk, intermittent or transient clonus.

DISCHARGE NOTE

ADMISSION DATE: Date admitted to hospital.
DISCHARGE DATE: Date discharged, scheduled or actual.
SERVICE: Pulmonology/Orthopedic/etc. Attending, residents.
REFERRING PHYSICIAN: Primary care physician, services.
CONSULTS: Physicians, specialties, dates, referrals.
PROCEDURES: Dates, Surgeries/Cultures/Imaging/etc.
HISTORY, PHYSICAL EXAM: Key admission data, lab results.
COURSE: Synopsis of treatments & progress during stay.
DISCHARGE CONDITION: Fair, Good, Guarded, Stable, etc.
DISPOSITION: D/C to home, skilled nursing, rehab, etc.
MEDICATIONS: D/C meds, doses, refills, and instructions.
INSTRUCTIONS: Diet, activity, dressings, report of findings.
FOLLOW-UP: Follow-up appt., who to call, providers, etc.

ELECTROLYTE IMBALANCES

	NORMAL	SX OF HIGH	SX OF LOW
K$^+$	3.5-5.0 mEq/L	↓HR, ↓BP, Paresthesias, Diarrhea, Prolonged QRS, Peaked T waves, Cardiac Arrest	Weakness, Cramps, ↓ Deep tendon reflexes, U waves, Resp. failure, Critical Arrhythmias
Na$^+$	135-145 mEq/L	Thirst, Seizures Restlessness, Muscle twitching	Confusion, N/V, Muscle weakness, Cramps, Seizures
Mg^{2+}	1.5-2.5 mg/dL	↓HR, ↓BP, Resp. depression, Cardiac arrest	Trousseasu's, Psychosis, Spasms, ↑Deep tendon ref.
Ca^{2+}	8.1-10.4 mg/dL	Muscle weakness, Altered LOC, Psychosis, ↓QT interval	Paresthesias, Trousseasu's, Osteoporosis, ↑QT interval
Cl$^-$	95-105 mEq/L	↑BP, ↑RR, Edema, Confusion, Weak, Headache	↓BP, ↓RR, Cramps, Disorientation, Hypoventilation
PO4	2.5-4.5 mg/dL	Paresthesias, Trousseau's, Osteoporosis, ↑QT interval	↓RR, Weakness, Cardiac depression, ↓Bone density

GLASGOW COMA SCALE

BEHAVIOR	RESONSE	SCORE
Eye opening	Spontaneously	4
	To speech	3
	To pain	2
	No response	1
Verbal	Oriented: time, place, & person	5
	Confused	4
	Inappropriate words	3
	Incomprehensible sounds	2
	No response	1
Motor	Obey commands	6
	Moves to localized pain	5
	Flexion withdrawal from pain	4
	Abnormal flexion (decorticate)	3
	Abnormal ext. (decerebrate)	2
	No response	1
Total score	Best response = 15 Minor brain injury = 13-15 Moderate brain injury = 9-12 Severe brain injury = 3-8	

HEIGHT CONVERSION TABLE

in	cm	cm	in
1	2.5	1	0.4
2	5.1	2	0.8
4	10.2	3	1.2
6	15.2	4	1.6
8	20.3	5	2.0
10	25.4	6	2.4
20	50.8	8	3.1
30	76.2	10	3.9
40	101.6	20	7.9
50	127.0	30	11.8
60	152.4	40	15.7
70	177.8	50	19.7
80	203.2	60	23.6
90	227.6	70	27.6
100	254.0	80	31.5
150	381.0	90	35.4
200	508.0	100	39.4

1 in = 2.54 cm	1 cm = 0.3937 in

HIGH ALERT MEDICATIONS

- **HIGH ALERT**
  - Heparin
  - Insulin
  - Potassium chloride
  - Opiates
  - NaCl > 0.9%

- **CAUTION**
  - Adrenergic agonists (e.g. dobutamine, epinephrine)
  - Chemotherapeutics
  - Chloral hydrate
  - Heparin
  - High-concentration dextrose > 10%
  - Hypoglycemic oral agents
  - Hypertonic NaCl > 0.9%
  - Insulin
  - IV adrenergic agonists (metoprolol, etc.)
  - IV digoxin
  - IV magnesium sulfate
  - IV potassium chloride/phosphate
  - Midazolam
  - Neuromuscular blocking (succinylcholine, etc.)
  - Opiates/opioids (fentanyl, morphine, etc.)
  - Warfarin
  - Topical anesthetics (Lidocaine, benzocaine, etc.)

HISTORY & PHYSICAL EXAM

- **CHIEF COMPLAINT**
  - o Health issue, patient's complaint in own words
- **HISTORY OF PRESENT ILLNESS**
  - o Timeline of events, location or body system involved, duration, frequency, severity, aggravating, alleviating, associated symptoms, self-treatment
- **PAST MEDICAL HISTORY**
  - o CURRENT HEALTH: date, type, outcome. CHILDHOOD ILLNESSES: measles, chicken pox, etc. ADULT ILLNESSES/INJURIES: hospitalizations, etc. IMMUNIZATIONS: polio, influenza, varicella, etc. SCREENING TESTS: pap smear, cholesterol, UA, etc.
- **PAST SURGICAL HISTORY**
  - o Type, dates, outcome, complications, transfusions
- **FAMILY HISTORY**
  - o Parents health/age/death, siblings, children, GENETIC: heart disease, diabetes, htn, cancer, mental illness, asthma, epilepsy, tuberculosis
- **MEDICATIONS**
  - o Type, dose, frequency, duration, compliance, access
- **ETOH, TOBACCO, DRUGS**
  - o Amount, frequency, duration, tolerance, pathology
- **ALLERGIES**
  - o Meds, foods, substances, swelling/breathing/rash

HISTORY & PHYSICAL EXAM

- **REVIEW OF SYSTMS**
  - GENERAL: fatigue, weight change, fever, chills
  - SKIN: hair, nails, itch, rash, sores, moles, lumps
  - HEAD: injuries, headache, nausea, visual changes
  - EYES: corrective lens, blurry, tearing, itching, loss
  - EARS: hearing change, tinnitus, vertigo, ache, pus
  - NOSE: congestion, sneeze, rhinorrhea, allergy, bleed
  - BREASTS: mass, lump, pain, discharge, skin, exams
  - CARDIAC: angina, htn, palpitation, murmur, dyspnea, orthopnea, edema, ecg/murmur hx
  - RESPIRATORY: wheeze, cough, sputum, x-rays, pna, short of breath hemoptysis, emphysema, asthma, tb
  - GI: n/v, dysphagia, appetite, hemorrhoid, stool color, melena, hematemesis, abd. pain, diarrhea, jaundice
  - URINARY: incontinence, frequency, dysuria, stones, urgency, infections, hematuria, polyuria, nocturia,
  - FEMALE GENITAL: period frequency/duration, STD, birth control, dysmenorrhea, pregnancies, sores, birth control, menopause, discharge, abortions, sex
  - VASCULAR: varicosities, edema, claudication, clots
  - MUSKULOSKELETAL: pain, weakness, joint stiffness, range of motion, redness, swelling, gout, arthritis
  - NEURO: tremors, numbness, weakness, faint, seizure
  - HEMATOLOGIC: petechiae, anemia, bruise, transfuse
  - ENDO: sweating, thyroid, diabetes, temp. intolerance
  - PSYCH: anxiety, depression, memory, mood, stress

HISTORY & PHYSICAL EXAM

HYSICAL EXAM
- **GENERAL:** sex/race, health status, stature, dress, hygiene
- **VITALS:** bp, hr, respirations, temperature, height, weight
- **SKIN:** rash, bruise, scar, hair, nails, tattoos, lesions, moist
- **HEAD:** symmetry, shape, size, scalp, lesions, trauma
- **EYES:** pupils symmetry/size/shape/reactive, conjunctiva, sclera, lids, extraocular movements, visual fields, acuity
- **EARS:** symmetry, shape, discharge, tender, tympanic membrane, auditory acuity, weber/rinne, inflammation
- **NOSE:** size, symmetry, tender, discharge, mucosa inflammation, frontal/maxillary sinus tenderness
- **MOUTH/THROAT:** dentition, tonsils, hygiene, patches
- **NECK:** range motion, thyroid size/nodules, trachea align
- **BREAST:** symmetry, tender, masses, dimpling, discharge
- **HEART:** rate/rhythm, murmur, S1/S2, gallops, rubs
- **LUNGS:** symmetry, wheeze/crackle, tactile fremitus, percussion, a-p diameter, diaphragmatic excursion
- **ABD:** appearance, bowel sounds, tenderness, soft/firm, masses, spleen/liver size, tympany/dullness, CVA tender
- **GU:** hernias, mucosa, inflammation, discharge, bleeding, bimanual palpation cervix/uterus/ovaries, scrotal mass
- **MUSCULOSKELETAL:** weakness/atrophy, motion range, swelling, tenderness, scoliosis/lordosis, gait, redness
- **VASCULAR:** edema, varicose, carotid bruit, pulses, JVD
- **LYMPH:** cervical, axillary, trochlear, inguinal, clavicular
- **NEURO:** sensation, strength, reflexes, cranial nerves, gait

IDEAL BODY WEIGHT

MALE:

- 106 + (6 x height in inches over 60")

Ex: 75-inch-tall male, IBW = 196 lbs.
      106 + (6 x 15)

FEMALE:

- 105 + (5 x height in inches over 60")

Ex: 67-inch-tall female, IBW = 140 lbs.
      105 + (5 x 7)

INTRACRANIAL PRESSURE SYMPTOMS

ASSESSMENT	EARLY SYMPTOMS	LATE SYMPTOMS
Level of consciousness	Restlessness/anxiety Speaking less Increased stimulation need Slight loss of orientation	Unarousable
Pupils	Sluggish reaction to light Unequal pupil size Unilateral pupil reaction Pupil Δ on side of lesion	Pupils fixed and dilated
Motor response	Acute onset weakness Motor Δ opposite side lesion One hand pronates when both held with palms up	Extreme weakness
Vital signs	Acute ↑BP fluctuations	↑SBP Wide pulse press. Bradycardia Irregular breath

INSULINS

TYPE	ONSET	PEAK	DURATION	FLUID
Regular	0.5-1 hr	2-4	6-8	Clear
NPH	1-2 hr	6-10	12 +	Cloudy
Aspart	< 10 min	1-2	4-6	Clear
Lispro	< 15 min	1-2	3-5	Clear
Glargine	1.5 hr	5	24	Clear
Lente	3-4 hr	4-12	12-18	Cloudy
Detemir	1.5 hr	5	12-24	Clear

LEAD PLACEMENT

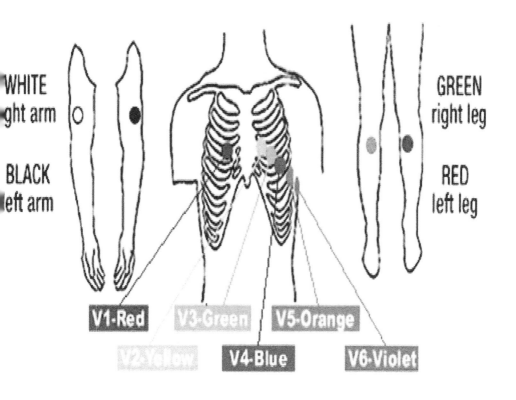

WHITE
ght arm

BLACK
eft arm

GREEN
right leg

RED
left leg

V1-Red

V2-Yellow

V3-Green

V4-Blue

V5-Orange

V6-Violet

LEVELS OF CONSCIOUSNESS

LOC	FEATURES
Lethargic	• Asleep often. • Awakens to verbal stimulation or gentle shake. • Stays awake with fare amount of stimulation.
Obtunded	• Severe drowsiness. • Awakens to forceful stimulation. • Remains awake for only minutes at a time.
Stuporous	• Very little movement. • Incomprehensible verbal response. • Awakens briefly to forceful stimulation.
Comatose	• No response to verbal or touch. • May withdrawal to painful stimuli. • Movement absent or non-purposeful.

LUNG VOLUME DESCRIPTIONS

PARAMETER	EXPLANATION
VT	Tidal Volume: Volume of air inhaled and exhaled during normal, quiet breathing
RV	Residual Volume: Volume remaining in lungs after maximal exhalation. RV/TLC ratio > 20% suggests obstructive disorder.
IRV	Inspiratory Reserve Volume: Maximum volume that can be inhaled after a normal inhalation.
ERV	Expiratory Reserve Volume: Maximum volume of air that can be exhaled after a normal inspiration.
TLC	Total Lung Capacity: Total volume of air contained in lungs. TLC=(IC+FRC) or (VC+RV) or (VT+IRV+ERV+RV)
VC	Vital Capacity: Maximum volume of air exhaled after a maximal inhalation. VC = (VT+IRV+ERV)
FRC	Functional Residual Capacity: Volume remaining in lungs after normal VT exhalation. FRC = ERV+RV. ↓ FRC and TLC = restrictive disorder.
IC	Inspiratory Capacity: Maximum amount that can be inspired after normal VT exhalation. (VT+IRV)
FEV1/FVC	Forced Expiratory Volume in first 1 second of FVC. Normal ≥ 80%. Obstructive < 80%.
FEF 25-75% or MMFR	Forced Exp. Flow (or Maximal mid-exp. flow rate) over middle 50% of FVC. Middle airway fx.

LUNG VOLUMES: OBSTRUCTIVE VS. CONSTRICTIVE

PARAMETER	RESTRICTIVE	OBSTRUCTIVE
TLC	↓	↑
VC	↓	↓
VT	N or ↓	Varies
IC	N or ↓	N or ↓
FRC	N or ↓	↑
IRV	↓	N or ↓
ERV	N or ↓	N or ↓
RV	N or ↓	↑
FEV 1 sec.	N or ↓	↓
FEF 25-75%	N or ↓	↓
MVV	N or ↓	↓
Peak Flow	N or ↓	↓

MAINTENANCE HOURLY FLUID

THE "4 – 2 – 1" RULE:
Hourly Fluid Requirements

- 4 ml/kg for the first 10 kg of a pt's weight
- 2 ml/kg for the next 10 kg of a pt's weight
- 1 ml/kg for the rest of the patients weight

Ex: 70 kg = (4 x 10)+(2 x 10)+(1 x 50) = 110 ml/hr

More simply... (Weight in kg)+(40) for pts ≥ 20 kg

MAJOR NERVES

NERVE	MOTOR	SENSATION
Axillary	Shoulder abduction	Lateral shoulder
Musculocutaneous	Elbow flexion	Lateral forearm
Median	Thumb opposition	Lateral palm
Radial	Finger extension	Dorsolateral hand
Ulnar	Finger ab/adduction	Medial hand
Obturator	Thing adduction	Medial thigh
Sciatic	Knee flexion	Posterolateral calf
Femoral	Knee extension	Anterior thigh
Peroneal	Toe extension	Dorsal foot
Tibial	Toe flexion	Plantar foot

MECHANICAL VENTILATION PARAMETERS

TERM	PARAMETER	FORMULA	NORMAL
V_T	Tidal Volume	V_E / f	5-10 mL/kg
V_E	Minute Ventilation	$V_T \times f$	5-10 L/min
f	Frequency or Rate	V_E / V_T	8-20 br./min
I:E Ratio	Insp.-to-Exp. Ratio	$T_I : T_E$	1:2 to 1:4
PIP	Peak Insp. Press.	$P_{Plateau} / R_{AW}$	< 40 cm H_2O
$P_{plateau}$	Plateau Pressure	$P_{Peak} - R_{AW}$	< 32 cm H_2O
P_{mean}	Mean airway press.	Manometer	5-10 cm H_2O
NIF	Negative Insp. Force	Manometer	> 80 cm H_2O
C_O	Dynamic compliance	$(V_T -$ tubing expansion vol.) $\div$ (PIP - PEEP)	Varies based on Cs and R_{AW}
C_S	Static compliance	$(V_T -$ tubing expansion vol.) $\div$ ($P_{Plateau}$-PEEP)	0.1-.2 cmH_2O
R_{AW}	Airway Resistance	$P_{Peak} - P_{plateau} \div$ flowrate L/sec	0.5-2.5 cm H_2O/L/sec
V_DMech	Mechanical Deadspace	10 mL/inch	0 if not using mechanism
V_A	Alveolar Ventilation	$(V_T - V_D) \times f$	Near V_E

MINI MENTAL STATUS EXAM

TASK	INSTRUCTIONS	POINTS
Date Orientation	"Tell me the date." Ask for missing info.	1 = each: year, season, date, day of week/month.
Place Orientation	"Where are you?" Ask for missing info.	1 = each: city, state, room, building, county, or room.
Register 3 Items	Name 3 items and ask pt. to repeat.	1 = each: object repeated correctly.
Serial 7's	"Count back from 100 by 7."	1 = each answer up to 5.
Recall 3 Items	Ask pt. to recall previously 3 items.	1 = each: item recalled correctly.
Naming	Point to watch and ask "What is this?" Repeat with pencil.	1 = each: correct answer.
Repeat a phrase	"No ifs, and or buts"	1 = success 1st try.
Verbal commands	"Take paper in R hand, fold in ½, put on the floor."	1 = each: correct action w/ paper given to pt.
Written commands	Show pt piece of paper with "Close your eye" written.	1 = if patient closes eyes.
Writing	Ask pt. to write a sentence.	1 = if sentence has verb, subject, & makes sense.
Drawing	Ask pt. to copy a pair of intersecting pentagons.	1 = figure has 10 corners & 2 intersecting lines.

Total possible = 30. Score ≥ 24 considered normal.

MORSE FALL SCALE

1. History of Fall in last 3 months	Yes 25 No 0	
2. Secondary Diagnosis	Yes 15 No 0	

3. Ambulatory Aid
  • Furniture
  • Crutch/cane/walker
  • Bed rest/nurse assist
	30
	15
	0	

4. IV/Heparin lock	Yes 20 No 0	

5. Gait/Transferring
  • Impaired
  • Weak
  • Normal/bed rest/immobile
	20
	10
	0	

6. Mental Status
  • Forgets limitations
  • Oriented to own ability
	15
	0	

Risk Level	MSF Score	Action
No Risk	0-24	Basic Nursing
Low Risk	25-50	Standard Fall Precautions
High Risk	≥	High Risk Fall Precautions

MURMURS

GRADE	DESCRIPTION
1	Barely audible
2	Audible, but soft
3	Easily audible
4	Loud, may produce palpable thrill
5	Very loud with light stethoscope pressure, thrill
6	Very loud, heard with stethoscope of chest, thrill

MUSCLE STRENGTH

SCORE	DESCRIPTION
0	No muscle contraction detected.
1	Visible muscle movement but not at the joint.
2	Movement at the joint but not against gravity.
3	Movement against gravity, not against resistance.
4	Movement against resistance but slightly limited.
5	Normal strength.

NERVE ROOTS

ROOT	MOTOR	SENSORY	REFLEX
C5	Shoulder abduction	Lateral arm	Biceps
C6	Wrist extension	Thumb, index	Brachioradialis
C7	Wrist flexion	Middle finger	Triceps
C8	Finger flexion	Ring, small	--
T1	Finger ab/aduction	Medial arm	--
L1	Hip flexion (T12-L3)	Ant./inner lower limbs	--
L2	Hip adduction (L2-L4)	Middle thigh	--
L3	Knee extension (Ls-L4)	Lower thigh	--
L4	Foot dorsiflexion & Inversion	Medial leg Medial foot	Patellar
L5	Toe extension	Lateral leg Dorsal foot	--
S1	Foot plantar flex & Eversion	Lateral foot	Achilles

ORIENTATION BEHAVIORS

ORIENTATION	BEHAVIORS
X 3	Understands verbal & written commands. Responds consistently.
X 2 **Mildly Confused**	Some difficulty w/ complicated commands. Occasional memory deficit. Gives approximate date or general time.
X 1 **Confused**	Difficulty following most commands. Frequently forgets. Cannot recall date or location.
DISORIENTED	Unable to follow any direction. May hallucinate or become agitated. Cannot answer appropriately or state name.

OXYGEN TANK FACTOR EQUATION & AIR ENTRAINMENT

Oxygen Tank Duration Calculation (minutes)

$$\frac{\text{Gauge pressure in psi X tank factor}}{\text{Liter flow (L/min)}}$$

Oxygen Tank Factors (L/psi)
- E cylinder = 0.28
- G cylinder = 2.4
- H cylinder = 3.1

Ex: Duration of E cylinder with 2200 psi at 4 L/M?

$$\frac{2200 \text{ X } 0.28}{4} = 154 \text{ minutes, or 2 hours \& 34 minutes}$$

Oxygen and Air Entrainment Ratios

FIO$_2$	Oxygen:Air
24%	1:25
28%	1:10
35%	1:4.3
40%	1:3
60%	1:1
70%	1:0.6
100%	1:0

OXYGEN DEVICES

DEVICE	RATE L/min	FiO2 %	NOTES
Nasal Cannula	1-6	24-44	FiO2= 24 + (2 x liter flow): 2=28%
Hi-flow NC	6-15	44-74	Heated/humidified, accurate FiO2
Simple Mask	5-8	40-60	Minimum 5 lpm to flush CO_2.
Venturi Mask	Vary	24-50	Precise FiO2. Must dial exact lpm.
Partial RB	8-15	60-80	Reservoir bag must be 2/3 full.
Nonrebreather	8-15	80-100	1-way valves stop CO2 rebreathe.
Oxymizer	1-6	28-46	>FiO2 than NC d/t reservoir.
O2 Conserver	1-6	24-44	O2 delivered only on inspiration.
Oxymask	1->15	24-90	Open mask for oral care. ≈ FiO2 ≈
Ambu bag	>15	100	Emergency use. Give 100% & Tv.

PACEMAKER CODES

LETTER POSITION	CATEGORY	CODE
I	Chamber paced	O = none A = atrium V = ventricle D = dual (A+V) S = single (A or V)
II	Chamber sensed	O = none A = atrium V = ventricle D = dual (A+V) S = single (A or V)
III	Pulse generator's Response	O = none T = triggered I = inhibited D = dual (T + I)
IV	Pacemaker's Programmability	O = inhibited C = communicating R = rate modulation M = multiprogrammable P = simple programmable
V	Anti-tachycardia Functions	O = none P = paced S = shocks D = dual (P+S)

PFT SPECIAL TEST DESCRIPTIONS

TEST	NORMAL	DESCRIPTION
DLCO	25 mL/m/mmHg	Measures diffusion across A-C membrane of carbon monoxide, helium, & air. Detects surface area defects when pt exhales into device.
FLOW-VOLUME LOOP	Volumes & flows predicted on age, gender, patho.	Volumes & flow rates of VC. Exhaling forcefully detects obstruction or restriction.
V/Q SCAN *or* VENT/PERFUSION		Gas/blood flow distribution. Inhalation of xenon & inject radio-isotope. Can show PE's & poorly ventilated areas.
HELIUM DILUTION	≤ 7 min Normal FRC	Calculates RV & TLC by measuring FRC. 10% helium breathed, measure time until equilibrium reached. Reveals obstruction longer it takes.
NITROGEN WASHOUT	< 8 min to reach < 2.5% N in lungs	Calculates FRC & RV by inhaling 100% O_2 & measuring time till N < 2.5%

PFT VALUES

PARAMETER	NORMAL	NORMAL 70kg
TLC (total lung capacity)	80 ml/kg	5600 mL
VC (vital capacity)	65 ml/kg	4500 mL
VT (tidal volume)	7 ml/kg	490 mL
FRC (function residual volume)	30 ml/kg	2100 mL
IC (inspiratory capacity)	50 ml/kg	3500 mL
IRV (inspiratory reserve volume)	40 ml/kg	2800 mL
RV (residual volume)	16 ml/kg	1120 mL
FEV 1 (forced exp. volume 1 sec)	60% FVC	3640 mL
FEF 25-75% (mid-flow rate)	4.7 L/sec	280 L/min
NIF (negative inspiratory force)	-80 cmH2O	-100 cmH2O
IS (incentive spirometer)	50 ml/kg	3500 ml
PF (peak flow)	500 L/min	600 L/min

POSTPARTUM & DELIVERY NOTES

DELIVER DATE/TIME

- **PHYSICIANS:** surgeon, attending, anesthesia
- **MOTHER:** age, race, gravida/para, group B strep +/-
- **ANESTHESIA:** spinal/epidural, pudental, local
- **DELIVERY:** spont. Vaginal, low transverse, C-section
- **INFANT:** weight, sex, APGAR 1 & 5 min, suction
- **UMBILICAL CORD:** nuchal, labs sent, 2 or 3 vessel
- **PLACENTA:** delivery time, intact, fragment, meconium
- **MEDS:** oxytocin, abx, cytotec, mag, methergine
- **CLOSURE:** sutures #, episiotomy, degree of laceration
- **ESTIMATED BLOOD LOSS:** amount in mL
- **COMPLICATIONS:** eclampsia, PROM, macrosomia
- **CONDITION:** mother & infant (stable, critical, etc.)

POSTPARTUM NOTE

- **S:** patient complaints, pain, breast tenderness, vaginal bleeding, urination, flatus, bowel, lower extremity swelling, ambulation, breast/bottle,
- **O:** VITALS: pulse, blood pressure, respirations, temp.
  I/O: emesis, urine, stool, IV fluid, PO, bleeding
  EXAM: fundal height/consistency, incision, edema, BS
  MEDS: pain, iron, laxative, RhoGam, vitamins
  LABS: rubella, Rh status, CBC
- **A:** assess findings w/ course of labor/delivery/recovery
- **P:** rubella immunization, meds, labs, discharge

PRELOAD/AFTERLOAD/CONTRACTILITY

	↑	↓
PRELOAD	- Volume gain (HF, ARF, IV fluids) - Vasoconstriction (↑venous return)	- Volume loss (bleeding, dehydration) - Vasodilation (↓venous return: shock, sepsis) - Tachycardia (↓ vent. fill) - Dysrhythmias
CONTRACTILTIY	- Volume gain - Inotropic meds - Catecholamines	- Volume loss - Negative inotropics - Hypoxia - Myocardial ischemia - ↓ Ca/Mg
AFTERLOAD	- Volume loss - Vasoconstrictor med - Cardiogenic shock - Hypertension - Aortic stenosis - Atherosclerosis	- Vasodilation drugs - Sepsis - Anaphylaxis - Fever

REOPERATIVE, PROCEDURE, & POSTOP NOTES

PEOPERATIVE NOTE
PRE-OP DIAGNOSIS: note any changes
PROCEDURE: surgery, general, sedation, laparoscopic, open
EKG/CHEST X-RAY/LABS: CBC, chemistries, PT/PTT, UA, etc.
BLOOD: type/screen, type/cross, # units, PRBC's, platelets, etc.
ORDERS: antibiotics, NPO, d/c blood thinners, bowel prep, etc.
CONSENT: signed/witnessed, in chart

OPERATIVE NOTE
PRE-OP DIAGNOSIS: note any changes
PROCEDURE: surgery, laparoscopic, open, robotic, positioning
SURGEONS: attending, residents, PA, consults, scrubbed
FINDINGS: ruptured appendix, peritoneal blood, etc.
ANESTHESIA: spinal, regional, general endotracheal (GETA)
FLUIDS: normal saline, lactated ringers, blood, amount
ESTIMATED BLOOD LOSS: amount mL
DRAINS: jackson, hemovac, suction, location, color, amount
SPECIMENS: tissue/organ, pathology, culture, etc.
COMPLICATIONS: laryngospasm, hemorrhage, anaphylaxis
CONDITION: stable, guarded, ICU, recovery, telemetry, d/c

POSTOPERATIVE NOTE
PROCEDURE:
S: patient complaints, pain, consciousness, etc.
O: Vitals, Meds (antibiotics), Labs, I&O (drains, IV, etc.)
A: based on data
P: consults, labs, meds, procedures, discharge

PRESSURE ULCERS

STAGE	FEATURES	INTERVENTIONS
I	Intact skin, painful, firm, cooler or warmer than surrounding skin, nonblanchable erythema	No dressing, protect from friction and shear forces, monitor regularly, relieve pressure, monitor frequently
II	Partial-thickness loss of epidermis or dermis, appears as abrasion, blister or shallow crater w/o slough or bruising	Dressing to keep bed evenly moist, keep surrounding skin intact & dry, loosely pack wound bed to remove excess moisture and for protection
III	Full-thickness, eschar & necrosis, subcutaneous tissue involvement, deep crater w/o undermining	Dressing to keep bed moist, surrounding tissue dry/intact, debride eschar/necrotic tissue surgically, wet-to-dry dress, mechanically, or irrigation
IV	Full-thickness, eschar, slough, necrosis, damage to muscle/bone, sinus tracts & undermining	Dressing to keep bed moist, surrounding tissue dry/intact, remove necrosis, explore undermining, control bleeding after sharp debridement then resume moist dressings

RESPIRATORY PATTERNS DIAGRAM

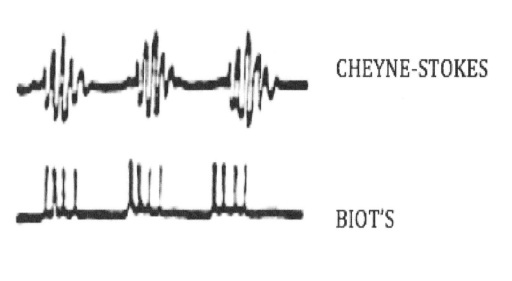

CHEYNE-STOKES

BIOT'S

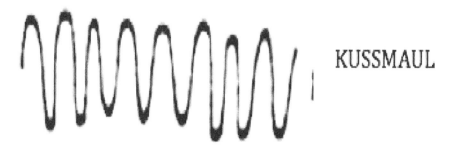

KUSSMAUL

SERUM DRUG LEVELS

DRUG	PEAK	TROUGH
Amikacin (amikin)	25-35 mcg/mL	< 10 mcg/mL
Gentamicin (gentamicin)	4-6 mcg/mL	< 2 mcg/mL
Tobramycin (nebcin)	4-6 mcg/mL	< 2 mcg/mL
Vancomycin (vancocin)	20-40 mcg/mL	< 10 mcg/mL

DRUG	THERAPEUTIC	TOXIC
Acetaminophen (tylenol)	5-20 mcg/mL	> 200 mcg/mL
Amiodarone (pacerone)	0.5-2 mcg/mL	> 2.5 mcg/mL
Carbamazepine (tegretol)	4-12 mcg/mL	> 12 mcg/mL
Digoxin (lanoxin)	0.8-2 mcg/mL	> 2 ng/mL
Ethosuximide (zarontin)	40-100 mcg/mL	> 150 mcg/mL
Lidocaine (xylocaine)	1.5-6 mcg/mL	> 6 mcg/mL
Lithium (lithobid)	0.6-1.2 mEq/L	> 1.5 mEq/L
Phenobarbital	15-40 mcg/mL	> 35 mcg/mL
Salicylate (aspirin)	10-30 mg/dL	> 40 mg/dL

STROKE SCALE: CINCINNATI

FEATURE	NORMAL	ABNORMAL
FACIALE DROOP	Both sides of face move equally	One side of face does not move at all
ARM DRIFT	Both arms move equally	One arm drifts compared to other arm
SPEECH	Uses correct words with no slurring	Slurred or inappropriate words or mute

TEMPERATURE CONVERSION TABLE

DEGREES FAHRENHEIT	DEGREES CELSIUS
95.0	35.0
95.4	35.2
96.2	35.7
96.8	36.0
97.2	36.2
97.6	36.4
98.0	36.7
98.6	37.0
99.0	37.2
99.3	37.4
99.7	37.6
100	37.8
100.4	38.0
100.8	38.2
101	38.2
101.2	38.4
101.4	38.5
101.8	38.8
102.0	38.9
103.0	39.4
(F − 32) ÷ 1.8 = Celsius	(C x 1.8) + 32 = Fahrenheit

TRANSFUSION REACTIONS

REACTION	SIGNS & SYMPTOMS	TREATMENT
Allergic	Dyspnea, wheezing, stridor, hives, loss of consciousness, shock, flushing, cardiac arrest	Antihistamines, steroids, ranitidine, epinephrine, vasopressin
Febrile non-hemolytic	Fever, chills, rigors, No dyspnea or ↓BP	NSAID, benadryl, leukocyte-reduced blood in future
Acute hemolytic	Fever, chill, itching, chest pain, anxiety, dyspnea, ↓BP, ↑HR, flushing, shock	Antihistamines, steroids, ranitidine, epinephrine, admit to ICU, resp. support
Contamination +/- Sepsis	Fever, chills, rigors, dyspnea, ↓BP, ↑HR	Blood cultures, abx, steroids, fluids, vasopressors
Acute lung injury	Dyspnea, cyanosis, hypoxia, ↓BP, ↑HR	O2, fluids, epi/vaso, ventilatory support
Circulatory overload	SOB, hypertension	O2, IV diuretics

TRANSFUSION TIMES

PRODUCT	TRANSFUSION TIME
Packed Red Blood Cells (PRBC)	1.5 – 2 hrs. Max 5 hrs.
Platelets	15-30 min. or as rapidly as tolerated Max 4 hrs.
Fresh Frozen Plasma (FFP)	10-20 min. or as rapidly as tolerated Max 4 hrs.
Cryoprecipitate	10-30 min., or as rapidly as tolerated Max 4 hrs.

TRANSLATION: ENGLISH TO SPANISH

ENGLISH	SPANISH
Angina	La angina
Appendicitis	La apendicitis
Asthma	El asma
Burn	La quemadura
Cancer	El cancer
Cold	El catarro, el resfriado
Constipation	El estreñimiento
Cough	La tos
Diabetes	La diabetes
Diarrhea	La diarrea
Discharge	El flujo
Dizziness	El vértigo, el mareo
Fatigue	La fatiga
Fever	La fiebre
Food poisoning	El envenenamieto por comestibles
Fracture	La fractura
Gallstone	El cálculo biliar
Headache	El dolor de cabeza

CONTINUED....

TRANSLATION: ENGLISH TO SPANISH

ENGLISH	SPANISH
Heart attack	El ataque al corazón
Heart burn	Las agruras, acedia
Heart disease	La enfermedad del corazón
Hepatitis	La hepatitis
Hernia	La hernia
Herpes	La herpes
Ill	Enfermo(a)
Infection	La infección
Injury	El daño la lastimadura
Itch	La picazón, la comezón
Lesion	La lesión, el daño
Lice	Los piojos
Lump	El bulto
Measles	El sarampión
Mumps	Las paperas
Obese	Obeso
Pain	El dolor
Palpitation	La palpitación

CONTINUED…

TRANSLATION: ENGLISH TO SPANISH

ENGLISH	SPANISH
Pneumonia	La pulmonia
Rash	La roncha, la salpullido
Rubella	La rubéola
Sore	La llaga
Sprain	La torcedura
Stomach ache	El dolor del estómago
Swelling	La hinchazón
Syphilis	La sífilìs
Tachycardia	La taquìcardia
Tooth ache	El dolor de muela
Tuberculosis	La tuberculosis
Unconsciousness	Pérdida del conocimiento
Vomit	El vómito
Wound	La herida
ENGLISH PHRASE	**SPANISH**
I will give you injection.	Quiseira darle a Ud un(a) inyección.
" " rectal medication	" " medicamento por el recto.
" " some pills.	" " píldoras.
" " a liquid medication.	" " medicamento en forma liquida.

CONTINUED...

TRANSLATION: ENGLISH TO SPANISH

ENGLISH PHRASE	SPANISH
This is how you take this medication.	Así se toma este medicamento
Do you take any medications?	Toma Ud. medicamentos?
How often do you take them?	Con qué frecuenca los toma?
What is the dosage for each medication that you take?	Cuál es la dosis para cada uno de los medicamentos?
Are you allergic to any medications?	Está Ud. alérgico a algúnos medicamentos?
Ask for help before getting up.	Llame anetes de levantarse.
Are you in pain?	Tiene dolor?
Do you feel lightheaded?	Se siente mareado?
Hello, my name is____ and Ill be your nurse.	Hola, me llamo ____ y soy su enfermera(o).
Do you want to use the restroom?	Quiere ir al báno?
Are you hungry/thirst?	Tiene hambre/sed?

CONTINUED

TRANSMISSION BASED PRECAUTIONS

PRECAUTION	INTERVENTIONS
Contact	- Place patient in private room. - Wear gloves whenever in patient's room and change gloves after contact. Remove gloves before leaving room. Wash hands frequently. - Wear fluid-resistant gown in room if body fluid contact anticipated. Remove when leaving room. - Limit patient transport/movement out of room.
Droplet	- Place patient in private room. - Wear mask when within 3 feet of patient. - Instruct visitors to wear masks within 3 feet. - Limit patient transport/movement out of room. - If pt. leaves room, must wear surgical mask.
Airborne	- Place patient in private room. - Room needs negative air pressure, door closed. - Disposable N-95 respirator worn if in room. - Limit patient transport/movement out of room. - If pt. leaves room, must wear surgical mask.

URINALYSIS

PARAMETER	NORMAL
pH	4.6 – 8.6
Protein	< 20 mg/dL
Specific gravity	1.01 – 1.03
Glucose	Negative
Ketones	Negative
Hemoglobin	Negative
Bilirubin	Negative
Albumin	0.01-0.1 g/24hr
Urobilinogen	< 1 mg/dL
Nitrite	Negative
Leukocyte esterase	Negative

VITAL SIGNS, WEIGHT, HEIGHT: BY AGE

AGE	lbs.	kg.	in.	cm.	HR	RR	SBP
Preterm	4	2	18	41	140	40-60	50-60
Term	7.5	3.5	21	53	125	40-60	60-70
6 mo	15	7	26	66	120	24-36	60-120
1 yr	22	10	31	79	120	22-30	65-125
3 yr	33	15	39	96	110	20-26	100
6 yr	44	20	46	117	100	20-24	100
8 yr	55	25	50	127	90	18-22	105
10 yr	66	30	54	137	90	18-22	110
11 yr	77	35	57	145	85	16-22	110
12 yr	88	40	60	152	85	16-22	115
14 yr	99	45	64	163	80	14-20	115

WEIGHT CONVERSION TABLE

POUNDS	KILOGRAMS
10	4.5
20	9
30	13.6
40	18.1
50	22.7
60	27.2
70	31.8
80	36.3
90	40.9
100	45.4
120	54.4
140	63.5
160	72.6
180	81.6
200	90.8
220	100
250	113.6
300	136.4
Kg = lbs. $\div$ 2.2	lbs. = kg x 2.2

WOUND CARE

PRODUCT	FEATURES	INDICATIONS	CONSIDERATIONS
Transparent Films	Semipermeable Waterproof O2 permeable Moist healing Germ barrier	Stage I & II Superficial Blisters Tears	Transparency allows visual inspection. Δ 2-3x/week. Doesn't absorb.
Hydrogel	H20/glycerin-infused gauze. Moist healing Wet-to-dry debridement	Stage II, III, & IV wounds	Need 2° dressing Reduces pain Δ once daily Doesn't absorb
Hydrocolloid	Occlusive & adhesive wafer. Rehydration Debridement of dry/necrotic	Stage II & III Granulating wounds w/ low-mod exudate	Easy application Reduces pain Residue/odor from breakdown Δ 2-3x/week
Alginate	Soft seaweed fibers. Absorbs up 20x weight	Stage III & IV w/ mod-high drainage	Need 2° dressing Comes in ribbons Δ once daily
Foam	Very absorbent Adhesive foam	Stage III & IV Heavy drain	Comfortable Δ 1-2/week
Antimicrobial w/silver	Inhibit bacteria Absorbent	Infected w/ ↑ exudate	Ø Prolonged use Iodine sensitivity

THANK YOU FOR STUDYING WITH US!

NURSEMASTERY.COM

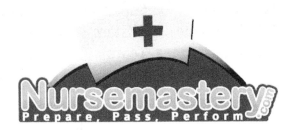

CHECKOUT:

- *"NCLEX REVIEW" APP*
- *1000 NCLEX QUESTIONS eBOOK*
- *SIGN UP FOR QUESTION OF THE DAY*
  - *twitter*
  - *youtube*
  - *facebook*

FREE GIFT!

At NurseMastery.com/downloads

or

Click the link for over 75 free NCLEX questions:

LINK TO FREE NCLEX QUESTION PDF

Made in the USA
Monee, IL
17 February 2024

53654994R00069